Diabetes:

*The Most Effective Methods to Defeat Diabetes
Once and For All. Quit Going to the Doctor, Quit
Wasting Money on Meds*

Alex Logan

Table of Contents

Introduction

Congratulations on downloading this book and thank you for doing so.

This book will give you a look into how traditional methods of treating diabetes, used by doctors everywhere, are actually not helpful and are often, indeed, even harmful to patients. We will talk about how these medications affect the body, and about alternatives that are being used to combat diabetes, in order to break the habit of dependence on doctors and lessen the impact of harmful medications on diabetics. You will learn how to control your diabetes using natural methods, how to live a better life, how to protect your body, and how to take control back from diabetes.

There are plenty of books on this subject on the market, thanks again for choosing this one! Every effort was made to ensure it is full of as much useful information as possible, please enjoy!

Chapter 1: What Is Diabetes?

Before we can get started on all of the information about controlling your diabetes, it is important to understand exactly what diabetes is and how it works. To this end, we will go over how the body normally processes sugar, the types of diabetes, terms that are used when talking about diabetes, and how diabetes affects the body.

Diabetes is, basically, the body having trouble processing glucose. Glucose is necessary for the body to function properly. It gives energy to cells throughout the body, and is produced by eating carbohydrates and other types of foods. When you eat these foods, your body breaks them down, and the resulting sugars are carried in your bloodstream through your body. Any glucose that your body does not use is stored mainly in your liver, but also in other tissue such as muscle, in the form of glycogen.

Hormones such as insulin, glucagon, and others help to regulate blood sugars. Their levels rise and fall to keep your blood sugars in a normal range. Too little or too much of these hormones can cause blood sugars to rise, resulting in hyperglycemia, or fall too low, resulting in hypoglycemia.

How does the body regulate blood sugar?

Normally, when you eat a meal, your blood sugar levels rise. When the glucose in your system rises, your system needs to take care of all that extra sugar, and so cells called "beta cells" in your pancreas release insulin. Insulin works to allow your body to absorb some of the glucose in the blood, making the blood glucose level fall back to normal. When your blood glucose level falls too low, the amount of insulin in your system lowers as well, and other cells in your pancreas release glucagon. Glucagon causes your liver to turn the sugar it's stored in the form of glycogen back into glucose, and release it into your bloodstream, causing your glucose levels to rise back to normal again.

How Insulin Works

Insulin, as mentioned above, is produced in your pancreas, and is the main player in controlling blood glucose levels. When you eat something that causes your blood sugar level to rise, your pancreas releases insulin. Insulin attaches to cells that can be used to store excess sugar for later, and signals them to allow the sugar in. Insulin is often thought of as a "key"; without it, cells do not know to open up and receive the sugar, and so the sugar stays in your system and results in high blood sugar.

Leptin

Other than insulin, a key player when it comes to blood sugar regulation is the hormone leptin. Leptin has an important part in whether or not a person will develop diabetes, as well. It is a hormone that is produced in cells like fat cells, and one of the main things it does is help your body manage your weight and appetite. It tells your brain when you need to eat, how much you need to eat, and when you should stop eating because you are full. It also signals your brain what to do with the energy that becomes available to your body through food. As stated above, when your body's blood sugar level rises, insulin is released by the pancreas to tell your body what to do with the extra sugar. Generally, it directs your body to store excess sugar in other cells, and one type of storage is in the fat cells. Leptin is produced in your fat cells. This is how the system works in a body that doesn't suffer from diabetes. It is a system of checks and balances, and it works very well to keep your energy levels where they should be and keep you feeling good. The problem of diabetes arises when this system does not work as it should. Before we go over the way the blood glucose level looks in a diabetic person, we should define some terms.

The Types of Diabetes and What Causes Them

If you have ever read anything about diabetes, or talked to anyone with the disease or any healthcare professional, you will likely be familiar with the terms "type 1" and "type 2" used to describe it. It's important to know the difference between type 1 and type 2 diabetes.

Type 1

Previously called juvenile diabetes, type 1 is generally diagnosed in children and young adults the most, though that is changing due to improper treatment of type 2 diabetes, which we will talk about later in this book. Type 1 diabetes is when your pancreas does not produce the insulin it should, leading to a lack of insulin in the body. Since insulin is used to regulate blood sugar, this leads to elevated glucose levels. The lack of insulin happens when your immune system destroys the cells that produce insulin, in your pancreas. It is also possible for people to have this type of diabetes without having had their immune system attack their pancreas. It can be caused by injury to the pancreas resulting in lower insulin production, or other diseases that can affect the pancreas.

If the pancreas does not release insulin, there is no hormone to tell your body to absorb the sugars that you eat. Instead, the glucose builds up in your system and the cells that should have been absorbing the glucose for energy starve. This causes high blood sugar, and type 1 diabetes.

Type 2

Type 2 diabetes also used to be known as adult-onset or noninsulin-dependent diabetes, and it affects the way your body processes sugar. It either resists the effects of insulin, or it doesn't produce enough insulin in order to maintain your blood sugar level where it should be. Type 2 diabetes begins with insulin resistance, which is when your body resists the effect of insulin. This causes higher levels of insulin to be released into your system, and when the body doesn't respond to that amount, even higher levels are released. Eventually the pancreas, trying to keep up with this higher demand for insulin, starts to fail. Not only can the pancreas fail due to insulin resistance, it also increases the level of insulin in the blood, since the body is not aware of how much insulin has been released due to the resistance. This resistance can happen due to a response to the body's own insulin, but can also happen when insulin is administered in the form of injections. We will go over insulin resistance due to injections, and how they can in fact make diabetes worse, later in the book.

The causes of type 2 diabetes are more varied than type 1, mostly because it is not fully known exactly why the body begins to develop insulin resistance. It is said that being overweight, being inactive, drinking soda, consuming too much sugar, and being genetically predisposed to the condition are all factors to developing insulin resistance and later type 2 diabetes.

So, while a person without diabetes is able to process the sugars they eat and turn them into energy, a person with diabetes is not able to do that the way that they should. Rather than the insulin being released properly, in the case of type 1 diabetics, there is little insulin in the blood, which causes a buildup of glucose and a high blood sugar level.

Insulin Resistance

Insulin resistance is also a key factor when it comes to the development or triggering of type 2 diabetes. Rather than the body responding the way that it should to the insulin that is released, as in type 2 diabetics, it resists the effects of insulin and doesn't absorb it properly, or it doesn't produce enough insulin in general. The inability to properly process glucose in the body causes diabetes sufferers to experience a variety of symptoms.

Leptin Resistance

Leptin resistance also contributes to the development of diabetes, as it has a lot to do with weight gain, which has been shown to trigger diabetes. The more fat you have, the more leptin you produce. When the sugar that has been directed to your fat cells is metabolized by those cells, they release more leptin into your system. Leptin is, in large part, responsible for whether or not you become insulin resistant. If there is too much leptin in your system, you can become leptin resistant, which means that your brain is no longer receiving proper signals about when to start and stop eating, and how much to eat. This can lead to chronic hunger, overeating, and an inability to burn fat properly, which can lead to obesity. Insulin resistance then follows suit.

Symptoms

It is important to keep an eye out for symptoms of diabetes, though if you're reading this book there is a good chance you have already been diagnosed. However, if you're unsure, here is a rundown of what both type 1 and type 2 diabetes look like.

Type 1 Symptoms

Given that type 1 is often diagnosed in children, it is important for parents and caretakers to watch for signs and symptoms of diabetes. These can include things that are more obvious, such as unintended weight loss, blurry vision, fatigue, and weakness. However, some of the symptoms are less obvious, especially in children who may be less apt at communicating their physical state. These can include bedwetting in a child who previously did not have that problem, marked thirst, extreme hunger, frequent urination, and irritability or other mood swings.

Type 2 symptoms

The symptoms of type 2 diabetes can often develop slowly. In fact, you may suffer from diabetes and be unaware of it for years. To avoid unnecessary discomfort and poor health, and get on the path to managing your diabetes, be on the lookout for these symptoms: increased thirst or hunger, weight loss, trouble healing cuts or bruises, dark patches on the skin, weakness, fatigue, and blurred vision. The symptoms of both types of diabetes are very similar, but they may look different in children and adults, so it's important to keep an eye out.

Insulin Resistance Symptoms

It is important to understand that insulin resistance often precedes the development of diabetes, so you should also be aware of the symptoms of insulin resistance. These can include feeling like your head is foggy and you can't focus, having high blood sugar, feeling intestinal bloating and gas, feeling sleepy after meals, trouble losing weight, weight gain, increased blood pressure, depression, and increased hunger. While these symptoms don't necessarily mean your body has become insulin resistant, it is still smart to keep an eye out for these symptoms, especially if you lead a less healthy lifestyle or are genetically predisposed to diabetes.

While the disease can often seem as if it's beyond your control, there are things you may be doing that could be exacerbating the symptoms. Stress can make your symptoms worse, as well as the things you are eating. A lot of the health issues and discomfort that arise from diabetes can be managed and controlled with changes to diet and lifestyle, without relying on expensive medications and doctors. We will discuss later in the book ways to manage these symptoms without resorting to harmful medical practices such as insulin injections or medications.

Chapter 2: Traditional Methods of Treating Diabetes

Now that we have learned a little about how the body processes glucose, and how that process differs in a diabetic, we can move on to talking about how diabetes is usually treated.

There are different methods of treating and controlling both type 1 and type 2 diabetes, but the main goal of all treatments is to keep the blood sugar level within the range your body wants it to be. For most people, the goal is to keep your daytime blood sugar levels between 70 and 130 mg/dL (milligrams per deciliter), before meals, and no higher than 180 mg/dL after meals, usually checked around two hours after eating.

Maintaining a proper blood sugar level in the traditional, medical way requires several steps.

Firstly, in order to be aware of their blood sugar levels, both at the base level and before and after meals, the diabetic must regularly check their blood sugar, using a blood glucose meter. This meter, usually about the size of the palm of your hand, is fed small strips with a drop of blood on them, which it tests to check the blood sugar level. The meter will either have a small needle built in, or the diabetic will have another piece of equipment called a lancing device that often looks like a pen, with a button. When that button is pressed, a small needle shoots out of one end, where the diabetic has pressed either their finger or another suitable body part. The needle pierces the skin, allowing a small amount of blood to well up, which the person can then soak up with the test strip.

Once a diabetic person checks their blood sugar and sees that it is not within the range it needs to be, they need to take steps to rectify it. This often means that the person will have to inject themselves with insulin that they measure out of a small bottle and inject into themselves, usually into their thigh. It can also mean having a snack to raise blood sugar if the levels are low, or taking medication that has been prescribed to them by their doctor. It can also mean that they have to adjust their insulin pump.

Insulin pumps are another way that doctors enable patients to be able to receive supplemental insulin. The pump is a small machine that houses a reservoir of insulin, usually about the size of a cell phone. It is attached to a catheter by a small tube. The catheter is inserted into the patient's skin, usually on their hip, and the pump can be worn in the patient's waistband, pocket, or even in a special holster made specifically for insulin pumps.

The idea behind the pump is the same as that behind insulin shots: it is to help maintain proper blood sugar levels by increasing the amount of insulin in the body. However, insulin pumps act a little differently. The insulin administered with injections is usually a long-acting insulin, and is administered less often, mostly when the blood sugar levels are tested and shown to be off. Insulin pumps, however, work differently. They release a more constant stream of insulin into the body, maintaining what is called the basal rate, and it replaces the long-acting insulin many people used before they got their insulin pump. People who use an insulin pump also program it with the amount of carbohydrates they're eating, as well as their blood sugar at the time, and the pump releases what is called a "bolus" dose to cover the meal that the person is about to eat and keep their blood sugar levels where they should be, as well as correct the blood sugar levels if they're too high.

Treating Type 1 Diabetes the Traditional Way

While treatment of both types of diabetes require blood glucose monitoring and adjusting, traditional medical treatments of both types of diabetes are different. Type 1 diabetics who are looking to manage their diabetes the traditional way will work closely with their doctor or a team of doctors to create a diabetes management plan. This plan usually consists of taking insulin every day, following a meal plan, checking blood sugar levels often, and getting enough exercise. The insulin is administered, as mentioned above, through either several shots throughout the day, or with the use of an insulin pump.

A healthy, balanced diet is also important when treating type 1 diabetes, as it helps maintain more steady blood glucose levels throughout the day by spreading carbohydrates out, rather than eating too many sugars at once. The meal plan does not usually lay out specific foods or meals that the patient should eat, but rather outlines what kinds of foods the patient should be choosing, which ones they should stay away from, and when they should be eating. It will provide guidance for breakfast, lunch, and dinner, as well as scheduled snacks between meals.

However, even though methods such as meal planning and exercise are used when treating and controlling type 1 diabetes, the main method of control and treatment is through the use of insulin. Since the pancreas is no longer able to produce insulin, doctors correct problems with patients' blood sugars with insulin administered through needles or pumps, and the harmful effects of this will be discussed later.

Treating Type 2 Diabetes the Traditional Way

Treatment and control of type 2 diabetes seems to be a little more well-rounded than that of type 1 diabetes, as it, in theory, is less focused on medication and more an overall lifestyle change. This is because type 2 can be brought on by poor lifestyle choices. Even jf a person is predisposed to diabetes, their lifestyle choices often do the work of actually bringing on the disease, and very often, at the very least, make it worse than it otherwise would be. Therefore, when traditionally treating type 2 diabetes, doctors will tell patients that while medication is important, doing things like changing the types of food you eat, how much you eat, getting more exercise, and monitoring your blood glucose levels are all supposed to be just as important as medication, whereas with type 1 diabetes, the most important thing is the insulin.

Healthy Eating

Contrary to what many people seem to think, there is no one specific "diabetes diet" that is prescribed by doctors and adhered to by diabetics who wish to control their diabetes through watching their food intake. There are, however, key things to focus on. It's important to try to eat mostly high-fiber, low-fat foods such as fruits and vegetables, as well as whole grains.

Exercise

Also important is getting enough exercise, as well as the type of exercise you do get. Everyone needs enough aerobic exercise, and diabetic people are no different. People looking to help control their type 2 diabetes by working with a doctor will discuss the type of exercise they should do with their doctor. They usually aim for around 30 minutes of exercise a day, if not more, but should also keep in mind that exercise lowers blood sugar levels, so it's important to routinely check blood sugar when you make exercise a part of your diabetes management plan.

We have talked about how diabetes affects the body's normal blood glucose absorption and the ways that doctors will try to help patients treat this, but this is possibly the most important point we will talk about with regards to treatment: treating type 2 diabetes with insulin and medication. Later in the book we will talk about why using this kind of treatment is harmful to diabetics, and the ways in which diabetics can move away from traditional medical treatment and begin to manage their diabetes on their own in a more natural way, but for now we will focus on the treatment itself.

While type 1 diabetics are prescribed supplementary insulin to help control their blood sugar levels, type 2 diabetics are subjected not only to insulin shots, but also to other medications that are supposed to help. In fact, doctors will often prescribe a group of medications, so type 2 diabetics end up taking several pills or self-administering several shots throughout the day that are supposed to regulate their blood sugar, often on top of also taking insulin shots.

These medications can include meglitinides, metformin,

thiazolidinediones, sulfonylureas, and others, as well as insulin therapy, which can mean one of several different types of insulin, and each work in different ways.

There are many different types of medications that can be used for diabetes management, and many combinations of these medications prescribed by doctors. However, for the purposes of this book, we will cover only four of these medications.

Metformin

Metformin is usually the first drug of choice to treat type 2 diabetes. It works at the liver to reduce the amount of sugar that is released back into the bloodstream. It does not help patients who have type 1 diabetes or insulin-dependent diabetes, as it does not affect the amount of insulin in the system, but rather the amount of sugars that are allowed back into the system by the liver. Doctors will often prescribe this medication first, and often alongside other antidiabetic medications, such as sulfonylureas, as well as insulin therapy.

Sulfonylureas

There are several different types of sulfonylureas, and each type is paired with a different other antidiabetic medication, such as metformin or thiazolidinediones. These medications work by raising the level of insulin that is released by your pancreas.

Meglitinides

Meglitinides are a class of medications that are also paired with other antidiabetic medications, such as metformin. They also work to increase the amount of insulin that is in a person's body, in order to lower the blood sugar levels. These medications work quickly and do not stay in the system for very long, which means that a diabetic person who is prescribed a meglitinide will have to take it before every meal.

Thiazolidinediones

These medications, like the others, are often paired up, and do not seem to be given on their own, therefore continually adding to the number of medications that a diabetic with type 2 diabetes is supposed to take. There are different types of thiazolidinediones, and the different types are paired with different other medications, just like the way meglitinides and sulfonylureas. They work by lowering insulin resistance in muscle and fat, as well as reducing the amount of glucose that is released into the system by the liver. These medications are often prescribed when a patient has tried other medicines to help control their blood sugar, but they have not had the desired effect.

Chapter 3: Why Drugs Are Not The Best Option

Why drugs are not the best option to treat diabetes

Now that we know a little about these medications and the ways they interact with the body to either reduce the amount of glucose in the blood or raise the level of insulin produced by the pancreas, we can talk about why these drugs are harmful.

Insulin resistance, as was mentioned before, is when your body still makes insulin, but does not respond to it in the way that it should, so the blood sugar level stays high. The body, thinking there is not enough insulin in the blood stream, works the pancreas harder and harder to release more insulin from the beta cells. This leads to levels of insulin that are too high, as well as still having a high blood sugar level.

While some of the medications that are prescribed for type 2 diabetes work by lowering the level of sugar that is released by the liver, therefore lowering the amount of sugar in the blood, many of them work in the pancreas instead, causing it to release more insulin. If a lack of insulin were the problem, then more insulin would be the logical solution, and would have a beneficial effect on the blood sugar levels in the body. Unfortunately, that is often not the case with type 2 diabetics.

Problems with insulin

Too often diabetes is seen purely as a lack of insulin or as too much sugar in the system, and in both of those views of the disease, the rational response is to increase the amount of insulin. However, when the problem is actually insulin resistance or leptin resistance, these drugs can make the problem worse, especially in the long run.

As we've discussed, insulin resistance means the body is no longer responsive to insulin in the way that it should be, so the pancreas releases more and more insulin to make up for a perceived deficiency. When you couple already present insulin resistance with drugs that only serve to force the beta cells to produce more insulin, it puts the pancreas under a lot of strain. Often, the pancreas has been struggling to push out more and more insulin for years, sometimes even decades.

Ron Rosedale, a doctor who has specialized in insulin resistance and leptin physiology and who also authored a book on proper dieting for diabetes called The Rosedale Diet, says that using these drugs to increase insulin production in patients who are insulin resistant is like beating a racehorse near the end of the race. The horse may run faster for a short period of time, but soon the strain of having ran the race coupled with the stress of being beaten and having to go faster causes the horse to collapse.

The same thing happens with patients whose doctors prescribe them medications that force the pancreas to create more insulin. Eventually the pancreas is unable to keep up with the perceived necessity for higher and higher levels of insulin, and it fails. This is more and more often leading to patients with type 2 diabetes also developing type 1.

Another thing that can cause the pancreas to give out is the insulin therapy itself. Doctors have placed far too much emphasis on insulin as the main form of treatment and management of both types of diabetes, when really it is only completely necessary for people with type 1 diabetes, since their pancreas is not able to make as much insulin as their body needs.

Traditional medicine talks about diabetes only as a disease where the patient has high blood sugar, which is generally said to be typically your body's inability to produce enough insulin. However, as we've learned, that is often not the case with people who have type 2 diabetes. The problem is often not that the body doesn't have enough insulin, but that there is plenty of it, it is just not being recognized or used.

Doctors and patients are often under the impression that insulin injections are the main way to treat both types, which leads to people who should not be injecting themselves with extra insulin being prescribed insulin injections. When that insulin is introduced into the system of a person with insulin resistance, the body is not able to make use of it properly, and indeed does not even recognize it. So the pancreas continues to make more insulin, working harder and harder, and now there is much more insulin in the system than there should be, as well as the pancreas being run down. Eventually the pancreas can give out completely, just as is the case when medications are used that increase the amount of insulin.

When you consider that often, these medications are prescribed in conjunction with insulin therapy, you can begin to see why conventional medical treatments for type 2 diabetes often make things worse.

Harmful side effects from medications

Besides the way that these medications affect the insulin levels and the pancreas, they also have negative side effects on other areas of the body.

Metformin can cause such symptoms as nausea, vomiting, stomach pain, and diarrhea. Another more serious, though not quite as common side effect is a condition called lactic acidosis, which is a buildup of lactate in the system. This condition has symptoms like tiredness, weakness, trouble breathing, unusual muscle pain sleepiness, and a slow or irregular heart rate. Lactic acidosis requires medical treatment, and is considered a serious side effect of metformin. Metformin can also interact with other drugs you may be taking for other conditions. It can decrease the effectiveness of heart or blood pressure drugs, like diuretics and calcium channel blockers. It can also increase the levels of heart rhythm problem drugs in your system, drugs like digoxin, procainamide, and quinidine. It can also increase the levels of antibiotics and pain medications in your system.

Sulfonylureas also come with a list of side effects, some more serious than others. Patients taking sulfonylureas may experience hunger, skin reactions, upset stomach, and dark-colored urine. These can be troublesome enough, but another possible side effect of taking sulfonylureas is weight gain. Considering that many diabetes patients also suffer from obesity, and often their diabetes is in fact brought on by their obesity, it seems counterproductive that a side effect of a very commonly prescribed medication for type 2 diabetics is weight gain. Weight gain is shown to make diabetes worse and make it harder to control. It is especially important to remember that sulfonylureas are very often prescribed in conjunction with metformin and other medications, so not only are patients taking the risk of experiencing the side effects of the sulfonylurea, such as weight gain, they also can experience any and all of the side effects that come along with the other medications they are taking.

Meglitinides also come with a set of possible side effects, and again, are often prescribed alongside other medications, meaning that the side effects can be compounded. Patients taking meglitinides can experience joint pain, back pain, coughing, diarrhea, and a stuffy nose, and those are just the common side effects. Less common but still possible side effects are constipation, and feelings of tingling, numbness, burning, and dizziness, and weight gain.

The final type of antidiabetic drug that we talked about earlier is the category of drugs called thiazolidinediones. These drugs can have the most dangerous side effects of all the ones we've talked about. As before, it is also important to remember that thiazolidinediones are often prescribed alongside other drugs like the three listed above, so patients can experience the side effects from all of them. Side effects of thiazolidinediones can include hives, pain in your muscles, gaining weight, a sore throat, a runny or stuffy nose, and headaches. Those side effects are considered minor and common. More serious side effects that patients can experience include fluid retention that can lead to heart failure, trouble breathing, pain in your chest, swelling of your lips, tongue, throat, or face, and symptoms of liver problems, such as feeling nauseous, stomach pain, throwing up, yellowish skin, and dark urine.

Not all patients experience all of the possible side effects for a given medication, and in fact, some patients don't experience or notice any side effects at all. However, it would be irresponsible to completely ignore the possibility of these side effects, especially considering that many of them can exacerbate the problems that diabetic patients already face. The problems of weight gain, body pain and weakness

As I mentioned above, several of the medications that are commonly prescribed, and prescribed together, have the possible side effect of weight gain. It is well established that an unhealthy weight, obesity, can lead to or trigger diabetes, and that one of the very best ways to control diabetes is to follow nutritional guidelines and a meal plan, and to watch how much you eat, and when. If a patient is taking a medication for their diabetes and also are obese, that patient's diabetes management could be made more difficult by the possible side effect of weight gain. Even if the patient does not outright gain weight due to the medication, several of the medications listed can also make it more difficult for patients to lose the weight they have already put on, further increasing the difficulty of diabetes management.

In that same vein, many of the other side effects listed can make using other methods to manage diabetes more difficult. Exercise is a known, effective method of diabetes management. It helps patients to lose weight and maintain a healthy weight, but exercise also lowers blood sugar naturally, so it can be incredibly helpful to diabetic patients. However, many of the side effects listed above can make exercise difficult or almost impossible to do as often as the patient should. Side effects such as muscle pain, joint pain, headaches, back pain, and upset stomach all make a patient feel as if they would rather be in bed resting than out running or at the gym.

If the side effects seem to have the possibility of exacerbating the already difficult nature of diabetes, then the medications should be considered as only a supplement, or a last resort, but too often they are the first option tried by a doctor. Rather than focus on other methods of treatment that may be less harmful and may actually work better, especially in the long run, doctors seem to be all too happy to prescribe these medications to their diabetic patients, sometimes seemingly without even considering the source of their diabetes, and whether the medications will actually even help them at all. After all, if a lack of insulin is not the problem, why prescribe a medication that is used to release more insulin?

Is it worth it?

Not only are the side effects sometimes nasty and overall a detriment to a diabetic's health, studies have shown that these medications, and especially insulin therapy, may not be doing all that much to increase the lifespan of diabetic patients, or the quality of life. Dr. Rosedale has said that diabetes is generally seen as an example of accelerated aging due to the way too much insulin in the body wears down the body. He says that prescribing insulin to a patient who has insulin resistance should be considered malpractice.

It is not just Dr. Rosedale who believes this, either. In a study that was published in the issue of JAMA International Medicine from June 30, 2014, the authors concluded that insulin therapy may be doing more harm than good, something that Dr. Rosedale has said for about twenty years.

Co-author John S. Yudkin says that the benefits of diabetes medication and insulin therapy may not outweigh the negatives, especially for patients over the age of 50. He says that although insulin therapy can technically lengthen life, if patients feel like their quality if life is reduced by being on insulin, it will outweigh any benefits that could come from treatments.

As an example, the authors say that a patient with type 2 diabetes who starts insulin therapy at age 45 and is able to lower their blood sugar by 1% might get an extra 10 months of healthy life. However, a person who begins treatment for their type 2 diabetes at age 75, may only gain an additional 3 weeks of healthy life. For many patients, these few weeks of life may not be worth all of the hassle, pain, and side effects of undergoing insulin therapy and taking antidiabetic medications.

With all of those side effects possible, and all of the detriments that come along with a regimen of antidiabetic medications and insulin therapy, it is not hard to see why many diabetes patients are looking for ways to get away from conventional medical treatment! Doctors, too often, do not rely on anything but their medication. Sure, they may tell their patients that a healthy diet and regular exercise are very important additions to their management plan, but too often the medication is the plan and the other, very beneficial components are just a side note.

That need not be the case. It is possible to control your type 2 diabetes without all of that medication. The problem is not that your body is not making enough insulin, it is that you are resistant to it, so adding more insulin will only overwhelm your body. Doctor Joseph Mercola, New York Times bestselling author thrice over and author of a webpage dedicated to information about health, says that giving insulin to a person with type 2 diabetes is one of the worst things a doctor can do, since it serves to make insulin and leptin resistance worse over time. He says the problem is not too little insulin, so the solution is not more insulin, it is restoring insulin and leptin sensitivity.

There are ways to accomplish this without resorting to harmful medical practices, and they're often actually easier and less costly than traditional medicine!

Chapter 4: Managing Diabetes Without Medication: The Natural Way

Before we get into the methods used by naturopathic practitioners, it is important to understand exactly what is meant by this term.

Naturopathy is an alternative approach to medicine than the conventional approach. In the traditional approach to medicine, the practitioner who is treating a diabetic patient will follow a tried and true, established formula for treating diabetes that includes methods that focus mainly on monitoring blood glucose and then having the patient use medicines to balance it.

Holistic or naturopathic practitioners, on the other hand, focus on treating the whole person. They help empower patients to be able to create the conditions for their optimal health, treating and preventing disease and poor health in a way that benefits their whole body in the long term. A provider of alternative medicine will take an approach that is more personalized for the patient, and may include prescribing the patient a different type of diet, more or different exercise, methods for reducing their stress, and other lifestyle changes.

Naturopathic and holistic medicine providers are less focused on prescribing medication and getting the patient out of their office. They care more about the long-term effects of the things they recommend to their patients. A naturopathic provider wants to make sure that the things they prescribe to their patients will not only help them with their current issue, in our case, diabetes, but will improve their overall health, and, possibly most importantly, will not diminish their health the way that prescription medications so often do.

Naturopathic and Holistic Methods

There are different approaches that a practitioner of naturopathic medicine may use to help treat and control a patient's diabetes. Control can be accomplished using a mixture of changes in diet, increased exercise, and herbal supplements and vitamin supplements, as well as various other lifestyle choices. We will cover each of these main approaches to treating diabetes naturally in this chapter, and outline some ways that you can beat your diabetes at home, without the use of medication or insulin.

Diet

When we talk about a healthy diet as a part of a naturopathic approach to diabetes management, we do not always mean the same type of "healthy diet" that many people go on in order to lose weight. Those diets are often focused just on losing fat and getting to a target weight, not specifically on diabetes health, or even on health at all. Many fad diets are actually very bad for you in the long run, and as soon as you tire of the restrictions they place on you, your weight goes right back up. Diabetes patients require a different type of diet because they have different health needs than a person without diabetes or a person who is dieting just to lose weight.

Foods a Diabetic Should Stay Away From

Firstly, there are foods that a diabetic person should remove from their diet in order to begin reversing the progress of the disease and increase insulin sensitivity again. A basic rule of thumb is to remove anything that is processed, including processed sugars and meats.

Sugar

Try to remove any excess sugar from your diet. Refined sugar rapidly spikes your blood glucose level and makes your body work harder to get rid of it something that you're struggling pancreas does not need. Fruit juices, soda, and other sugary drinks are common culprits and should be avoided. Natural sweeteners like honey are better alternatives, but they can still cause a huge spike in blood sugar levels, so a good option is to replace your added sugar with stevia.

Refined foods

Highly refined foods are also to be avoided by diabetics. Refined foods are processed foods that have lost most of their vitamins and nutrients in the refining process, and they add a lot of calories to your diet compared to the benefits they give. The refining process is focused on carbohydrates like grains and sugars. They are refined to give the food a better taste and improve the product's shelf life. Refined foods often have more sugar in them as well, which relates to the point above.

Grains

Another culprit when it comes to a too-high sugar intake is eating grains. Even the healthy options like whole grains, organic grains, and sprouted grains all have a lot of carbs that are bad for a diabetic, as carbs are turned into sugar.

Diabetics should avoid bread, cereal, pasta, rice, and corn, which is actually a grain. Fiber is very important, but there are healthier ways to get enough of it, and we will go over them in a bit.

Processed meats

Studies have shown that eating processed meats is linked to a 42% higher risk of developing heart disease compared to eating only unprocessed meats, as well as a 19% higher risk of type 2 diabetes. Foods like deli meat, sausages, and hot dogs all have higher levels of sodium and preservatives in them, and should be avoided.

Trans fats

Trans fats are made when oils are turned from a liquid form into a solid form through the process of hydrogenation. It's easy to find trans fats on food labels even if the label says there are no trans fats, as they are allowed to say if the amount of trans fat in the food does not exceed .5 grams. The key word to look for is "hydrogenated", such as "hydrogenated oil" or "partially hydrogenated oil". You can find trans fats in many different types of food, such as prepackaged foods like snack cakes, muffins, potato chips, crackers and cookies, as well as in stick margarine and shortening. Research has shown that not only are trans fats bad for the heart, they can also be linked to insulin sensitivity.

Sodium

People with diabetes also often have high blood pressure. Salt can increase hypertension, or high blood pressure, and so should be avoided by diabetics. This is one of those things that naturalistic practitioners pay attention to when traditional medicine may not. It is not directly related to blood sugar or insulin, so things like this can be overlooked by doctors when discussing a diabetes diet. However, the diabetic body should be treated like a whole body, and keeping an eye on things like salt intake goes a long way toward making a diabetic person feel better, even if it doesn't involve their pancreas.

Foods a Diabetic Should Eat

While there may seem to be a lot of foods to cut out of your diet, there are also a lot of things you can and should eat a lot of. It may take some getting used to, but after your body gets used to consuming fewer refined sugars, carbs, and "bad" fatty foods, it will feel better than it did when you were eating that junk. The foods you should be eating as a diabetic are also delicious. You do not have to sacrifice flavor and enjoyment to follow a diabetic-friendly diet. Below is a list of foods you should be eating as a diabetic.

Protein

Diabetics should be eating protein at every meal. Protein helps to satisfy your hunger, so you are less likely to go for carb-filled snacks later. It also helps the body process sugar more slowly. If you are going to be eating carbs with your meal, the protein helps your body process that rush of sugars in a more controlled way, so it will not spike your blood sugar the way it would if you just had a bowl of pasta for dinner. Protein also contains good fats that you need for your body's overall health.

Fish

While fish also falls under the umbrella of protein, it is important enough to merit its own section. Fish is a very healthy protein that contains the omega-3s your body needs. Diabetic people can benefit a lot from additional omega-3s. Good fish choices for a diabetic are Albacore tuna, herring, rainbow trout, salmon, sardines, mackerel, cod, halibut, and tilapia. Also good additions to a diabetic's menu are other types of seafood, including clams, crab, scallops, lobster, oysters, and shrimp. Fish and other seafood can be a great way to incorporate protein in your meals without having to eat beef or chicken or some other heavier protein that you may not be desiring at the time.

Vegetables

You have been advised to cut out grains from your diet, and this may seem counterintuitive. After all, you know that you need fiber, and diabetics especially need fiber, so how are you supposed to get the fiber you need through your food if you are not supposed to eat grains? The answer: vegetables. Diabetics should eat as many low starch vegetables as they want, and some dieticians recommend sautéing the vegetables in butter, olive oil, or coconut oil to add "good" fats. So if you are craving some asparagus sautéed in olive oil with rosemary, or broccoli with garlic butter, go ahead and indulge! The fiber you get from these vegetables helps control your blood sugar and also helps fill you up. A diet high in fiber helps you feel more full, but also, because the body does not require insulin to process fiber, it helps keep your blood glucose level from spiking after you eat it. A part of the fiber stays intact and passes through your system. As an added bonus, fiber also helps keep your digestive system regular, and this kind of overall health focus is exactly what a naturalistic approach to controlling diabetes is all about.

"Good" fats

Recent studies show that diabetics should be eating "good" fats. These include monounsaturated and polyunsaturated fats. Many practitioners also believe that diabetics should be eating saturated fats, even though they have long been considered unhealthy fats. Dr. Mercola advises that diabetics eat saturated fats, based on a study that was done using dolphins. Researchers found that the dolphins were able to move in and out of a diabetic state, and also developed metabolic syndrome that then seemed to disappear.

Curious about how this was happening, researchers studied the dolphins and their eating habits, to see if their food could have something to do with the changes. They looked into the dolphins' diet and saw that a saturated fat called heptadecanoic acid was in their system, and it was lowering their insulin.

The type of food they were eating, in their case, fish, had an effect on their metabolism, and the dolphins that had that that kind of fat in their system had insulin levels that were lower. This study is being used to argue that saturated fats are also good for diabetics.

Saturated fat has been shown to have health benefits other than just reducing the amount of insulin in the body. These include helping with mineral absorption, helping to lower cholesterol levels, and providing building material for hormones, substances that are like hormones, and membranes around cells. Saturated fats also act as optimal fuel for your brain, carry important fat-soluble vitamins such as A, K, E, and D, and act as an antiviral agent.

You can get saturated fats into your diet by using coconut oil or avocado oil to cook with, and by eating butter, nuts, avocados, and animal fats.
Probiotics and Prebiotics

If you have paid attention to any yogurt commercial on TV, you likely know that probiotics are good for you and are found in many different foods. What you may not know is what probiotics actually are: bacteria. These bacteria help regulate the natural flora and fauna in your digestive tract. Prebiotics, on the other hand, are the foods that probiotics need to be able to do their job. It may seem strange to think of bacteria in your body, and may even turn your stomach at first, but these microorganisms are beneficial to you, and in fact, many already live inside you and do their part to keep you healthy.

Foods that are high in probiotics should also be included in a diabetic's diet. These foods include yogurt, kefir (a cultured drink that is similar to a drinkable yogurt), sour cream, buttermilk, aged cheeses such as Swiss and Gouda, cottage cheese with active cultures, miso, sauerkraut, and pickles. However, if you plan to intentionally consume foods that are high in probiotics, you should also plan to eat prebiotics, to provide fuel to the bacteria. Humans don't process prebiotics, so these nutrients pass through the system until they reach the large intestine, where they are used by probiotic bacteria. Prebiotic foods include asparagus, bananas, onions, leeks, garlic, and oatmeal.

What a Diabetic Diet Looks Like Day to Day

It can be daunting to change the way you eat. If you have been eating the same way for a long time, it can be hard to break unhealthy eating habits, because it seems like you are just denying yourself the things you want. In fact, if you have been consuming a lot of sugar, especially in the form of high-fructose corn syrup, your body can crave the sugar after you cut it down or cut it out completely. It can make sticking to a new diet hard.

With that in mind, I have included a few sample diabetes diet meal plans to help you get started creating your own. These can be tweaked to include foods you enjoy that are on the list of good-for-you foods, and to take out foods that you may not like. It can take some experimenting to find meal plans that work for you, but a good way to do that is to start with an outline or example and make it your own.

Sample Meal Plan One

Breakfast: One or two eggs prepared your favorite way (fried with butter is a good way to include saturated fat, and is also delicious), with nitrate-free, farm-raised bacon

Lunch: A big salad with carrots, onions, beets, tomatoes, black olives, cucumbers, and whatever other veggies you like in your salad. Add walnuts or pumpkin seeds, and goat cheese or feta. You can top it with a hard-boiled egg, grilled chicken, or tuna fish, and dress it with olive oil and vinegar.

Dinner: Halibut and an assortment of grilled or roasted vegetables. Try onions, carrots, and potatoes in the fall, and squash, peppers, onions in the summer. Alongside this, you could have brown rice.

Snacks: Four squares of chocolate with a high cacao content, with walnuts, cashews, almonds, or pecans. The sugar in the chocolate can help satisfy a sweet tooth, but choose chocolate with a high cacao content. Cacao is good for you, and chocolate that is high in cacao has less sugar, making it better for a diabetic. Also remember to eat nuts along with it, as the protein in them will help slow digestion of sugars from the chocolate.

Sample Meal Plan Two

Breakfast: A smoothie with 80% vegetables and herbs, and 20% fruit, with your favorite kind of nuts. Smoothies are a great breakfast choice as they can be eaten on the go, and are also a great way to get more veggies in your diet. Feel free to add some sweetener if it is not sweet enough for your taste; stevia is a good choice, but honey is also acceptable. You can also add some almond milk if you prefer a creamy smoothie.

Lunch: A collard green wrap with hummus, veggies, and avocado, and olive oil to dress it. Avocados are a source of good fats and are also very satisfying. Hummus is filling and the spiciness of it can help curb appetites.

Dinner: Chicken breast in a Thai peanut sauce over sautéed bell peppers and bok choy. Bell peppers and bok choy are great vegetable choices for diabetics, and chicken is a good source of healthy protein. Peanuts are also a good choice for a diabetic diet, as they are high in fat and omega-6.

Snacks: Fresh fruit and a handful of nuts. Be sure to be

careful how much fruit you consume, however, as too much sweet fruit can cause your blood sugar to spike. Bananas are a good choice, as well as apples, because the fiber in apples aids digestion, not to mention the fact that apples naturally help you feel more alert and energetic. If you eat fruit for your snack, do not forget the nuts to go with it. The protein in the nuts will help to slow the metabolization of the sugars in the fruit.

Sample Meal Plan Three

Breakfast: Oatmeal with honey, fruit, and nuts like almonds or cashews, and a glass of whole milk or almond milk.

Lunch: A small bowl of chicken and vegetable soup made with real bone broth, alongside a salad full of vegetables like cucumbers, tomatoes, spinach, romaine lettuce, olives, and topped with feta or goat cheese.

Dinner: A small burger made with all-natural, grass-fed beef, without a bun. You can top it with things like sauerkraut or pickles, as well as ketchup or mustard. Alongside this you can have vegetables like brussels sprouts, pickles, and tomatoes, as well as a half-plate salad dressed with olive oil and vinegar. Pickles and sauerkraut are a great way to incorporate probiotics into your diet.

Snacks: A half cup of yogurt topped with small amounts of fruits, nuts, and seeds. Yogurt is another great way to eat probiotics.

Exercise

Another very effective way of managing your type 2 diabetes, and indeed even type 1 diabetics benefit greatly, is with exercise. If you try to stay fit and active throughout your life, it will be easier for you to control your blood glucose level and keep it in the correct range. However, exercise will help not only your blood glucose level, but will also increase your insulin sensitivity, as well as your leptin sensitivity.

Exercise has many benefits for all different types of people, but especially for diabetic patients. Possibly the biggest benefit for diabetics is that exercise helps you control your blood glucose level. As we discussed in the first chapter, diabetics have too much glucose in their blood, either because their body does not produce enough insulin, or because it cannot use the insulin the way that it should because of insulin resistance. In either case, exercise can help reduce the amount of sugar in your blood. A major way this happens is that muscles can use sugar without the help of insulin when you are exercising. So it does not matter if you are insulin deficient or insulin resistant, because when you exercise, your muscles get the sugar that they need, and as a result the amount of sugar in your blood stream goes down.

The benefits are actually even higher for those diabetics who are insulin resistant. Exercise actually helps your body retain insulin sensitivity, making the insulin more effective and reducing insulin resistance. This also reduces the amount of insulin that the body thinks needs to be released into the system, which relieves some of the pressure that is placed on the pancreas to produce a lot more insulin than it should be.

Exercise can also be beneficial to diabetics in ways that are not directly related to sugar, insulin, or their pancreas. An active lifestyle can help patients with type 2 diabetes avoid other long-term health complications, especially heart problems. Many people who are diagnosed with type 2 are also overweight or obese, and exercising can help bring weight down to a healthy place, therefore helping to avoid health problems due to weight that can make managing diabetes even more difficult. Diabetics are susceptible to developing arteriosclerosis (blocked arteries), which can then end up in a heart attack. Exercise can help keep your good cholesterol level high and your bad cholesterol level low, helping to avoid heart attacks and keep your heart healthy and strong.

Additionally, there are all of the other health benefits to leading an active lifestyle. Your blood pressure gets lower, you get leaner, stronger muscles, your bones get stronger, you have more energy, you sleep better, your mood improves, and you're better able to manage stress.

All of these benefits are one of the reasons why it can be so much more helpful for a person with diabetes to approach management of their disease from a holistic, naturopathic viewpoint rather than from traditional medicine. Naturopathic practitioners aim to help the entire body, and while a doctor may tell a diabetic patient that exercise is important and should be included in their management plan, they may not talk about the way exercising benefits the whole body and the mind. They have a tendency to think only about the disease they are trying to heal, which leads to a narrow viewpoint and a limited management plan.

A doctor may tell a diabetes patient to do cardio to reduce weight, but may not tell that patient that other types of exercise are very beneficial, such as what is called "burst training", which is exercising in short bursts rather than long workout sessions, lifting weights, and doing more peaceful types of exercise such as yoga and pilates.

Burst training can be especially beneficial to diabetics, and studies have shown it may be even more beneficial than traditional 30 minute low-intensity workouts. As shown by research presented at the 2015 American Heart Association's Scientific Sessions, researchers found that people who had done three months of high-intensity 10-minute burst workouts three times a day had lowered their blood sugar an average of 82%, compared to people who performed more sustained, lower-intensity workouts, who only averaged a 25% decrease.

Part of the reason why burst exercising seems to work better is that it gets your heart rate up, faster. It also is easier to fit into busy schedules, which leaves less room for excuses that you did not have time or were too busy; it is much easier to fit in 10 minutes of exercise during the day three times than one big 30 minute chunk of exercise. High intensity bursts of exercise also change how well the heart functions, which is very important in a diabetic.

Diabetes is known to affect the heart; people with type 2 diabetes are often known to have changes in the heart's structure that affect the left ventricle, which gets blood from the left atrium and then pumps it out into the body. Research has found that high intensity bursts of exercise are able to improve the ability of the left ventricle to take in blood and make it more efficient. High intensity burst workouts are also said to improve blood sugar in that they help reduce the amount of fat in the liver, which can contribute to high blood sugar.

An example of a burst exercising workout on a stationary bike might look like this:

- Warm up for 3 minutes

- 30 seconds of pedaling as fast as you can. You should struggle to exercise for even a few seconds longer at the end of this stage, almost feeling like you cannot do any more.

- Rest and recover for 90 seconds.

- Repeat the alternations of high intensity pedaling and recovery period until you reach the end of the amount of time you want to work out.

Another type of exercising that is important for diabetics is strength training. As I mentioned before, your muscles can use sugar without the need for insulin, when you are exercising. So if you strengthen your muscles, you improve their function and ability to work longer and harder, and therefore use up more of the sugar in your system, which, of course, also lessens the strain on your pancreas having to produce more insulin. You can work on your muscles by doing things like lifting weights or using resistance bands, but you can also use your own body weight, by doing exercises like squats, lunges, and pull ups. You should aim to do strength training twice a week.

Yoga is another type of exercise that many people with diabetes have turned to. It has a lot of the same benefits as strength training, actually, but in a more relaxing package. Yoga poses require the person doing them to maintain the same position, meaning that their muscles develop strength the more that they do these poses, in order to keep them upright and balanced. As we discussed above, improving muscle strength can do wonders for blood sugar control. Yoga is also a stress reliever, allowing the practitioner a few moments of calm in an otherwise busy day. Stress has been shown to make diabetes worse. Stress is hard on the body in general, but also, people who are stressed often eat more, and often eat unhealthy things, which can spike the blood sugar. Less stress is an overall health benefit, but especially for diabetics.

It is important to note that before you do any type of exercise you should consult with a doctor, even if you are not using a doctor to help manage your diabetes in particular. While exercise is incredibly beneficial to your body, if you are already dealing with health issues, it can be dangerous. For example, a person with heart issues needs to be careful with cardio exercises.

Also, many people with diabetes struggle with obesity as well, and may not be physically able to do some exercises until they lose some of their weight and get to a more healthy place, so you may need to start slow and build up to the type of exercise you would like to be doing. Do not push yourself too hard too fast; exercise is supposed to make your life better, not worse, and the best way to insure that you will not make it a habit is to make yourself miserable while doing it. Try to find exercises you enjoy, consider taking a friend with you to the gym to keep you accountable and have someone to chat with.

Herbal and Vitamin Supplements

The final way to help control your diabetes without a doctor that we will discuss in this book is by using herbal and vitamin supplements. These supplements can help reduce your blood sugar, improve insulin sensitivity, and can also help improve your body in other ways, such as help you lose weight and help keep your organs healthy. Diabetes can be considered a wasting disease, as it leaches nutrients from your body. Elevated blood sugar acts like a diuretic and can cause a loss of nutrition in a diabetic's urine. Because of this, people who have type 2 diabetes often have deficiencies in water-soluble vitamins and minerals. Research suggests that people who have type 2 should, at a minimum, be taking some type of good vitamin and mineral supplement every day, as this has been shown to reduce the amount of infections a diabetic person gets, as well as sick days they must take due to not feeling well.

Specific supplements can be broken down into vitamins, minerals, and herbs. In this chapter we will go over a variety of each of these types of supplements, explaining why you should be taking them and what they can do for your body.

Vitamins

B-complex vitamins: Vitamins B6 and B12 are especially useful, as they support nerve health. This is important, since diabetic neuropathy is a real risk to a diabetic patient. Diabetic neuropathy is a nerve condition that can cause weakness, loss of sensation in hands and feet, digestive problems, carpal tunnel, and even erectile dysfunction. Biotin is another B vitamin that is important for growth and metabolism. You may be familiar with biotin as a vitamin that is recommended for people who are trying to improve the health of their hair, skin, and nails, as well as being recommended as part of a system of prenatal vitamins for expectant mothers. This is because biotin supports growth and metabolism, which can also help your body process sugars.

It is recommended to take 300 mcg of biotin, 150 mcg of B12, and 75 mg of B6 every day.

Vitamin D: This is another vitamin that is especially important to diabetics. Doctors have recently been linking type 2 diabetes with a vitamin D deficiency. Patients who were diagnosed with type 2 diabetes were shown to have very low levels of vitamin D in their systems. Doctors believe this may be because vitamin D helps "switch on" the beta cells in the pancreas, and those cells are the ones that produce insulin. If a person does not get enough vitamin D, those cells may not be working to their full potential. Vitamin D is also being said to help improve insulin sensitivity.
It is recommended to take 2,000 IU of supplemental vitamin D, at least, every day.

Vitamin C: Vitamin C lowers the level of sorbitol in your system, which is a sugar that can be bad for your eyes, kidneys, and nerves; if it is allowed to collect there, it can damage them. It is recommended to take at least 3,000 mg of vitamin C daily.

Vitamin E: Another alphabetic vitamin that is very important is vitamin E, and it is vital for all people regardless of health status. Vitamin E is the body's main fat-soluble antioxidant, which means it is very important. It helps to improve blood sugar control and protects nerves and blood vessels from damage from free radicals, which diabetes makes worse. Studies have even shown that vitamin E may reverse nerve damage due to diabetes.

It is recommended that you take 200 IU of vitamin E every day, whether you have diabetes or not. However, be sure to take only the natural form of it, which will be listed as d-alpha-tocopherol or d-alpha-tocopheryl.

Minerals

Chromium: Perhaps the most important mineral a diabetic could take, chromium actually helps your body use insulin better. It does not cause the pancreas to produce more insulin, just allows your body to more effectively use what is already there. Chromium has been shown to lower insulin resistance in patients with diabetes in over 15 studies.

It is recommended that you take 200-400 mcg of chromium picolinate daily.

Magnesium: Another very important and well known mineral for the management of diabetes, magnesium is vital for protein synthesis and energy production, as well as DNA production and cellular replication. Magnesium also helps improve insulin sensitivity.

It is recommended that you take 500-1,000 mg of magnesium daily.

Omega-3 fatty acids: We talked about omega-3s earlier when we were discussing diet, but you can also get the omega-3s you need from supplements. It is recommended that you take fish oil pills as an easy way to get your omega-3s, in addition to the omega-3s you get by eating healthy foods like fish. Take the recommended dose of the brand you choose.

Herbs

Cinnamon: An easy one to incorporate into your diet, cinnamon has many health benefits and has been used around the world for centuries as a holistic medicine. It is good for your heart and blood health, and can lower blood sugar levels. You can sprinkle it on your food, especially your oatmeal in the morning, so it's easy to get it into your diet. Make sure it is the unsweetened kind, however.

Purslane: Generally considered in the US to be a weed, but enjoyed in Europe and Asia, purslane is a plant that can help control blood glucose. The purslane extract Portusana enhances glucose uptake, slows the movement of glucose into your blood, and increases your insulin sensitivity. 180 mg a day is a generally recommended dose.

Pterocarpus marsupium: Also known as Indian kino tree extract, pterocarpus marsupium is extracted from the wood and bark of a tree that people have been using in India for a very long time in the traditional medical field. The flavonoids in it promote insulin sensitivity, improve your body transport sugar from your bloodstream into cells, and help manage blood sugar levels. 450 mg of a standardized extract daily is the recommended dose.

Bitter melon: Though it may sound like a fruit, bitter melon is actually a plant and can be found in supplement form. There is evidence that it may help in reducing blood sugar levels, and it is generally safe for everyone, which makes it a favorite. 900 mg is a good starting dose.

Conclusion

Thank for making it through to the end of this book, let's hope it was informative and able to provide you with all of the tools you need to achieve your goals whatever they may be.

In this book you have learned exactly what diabetes is. You now know the difference between type 1 and type 2 diabetes. You know that type 1 diabetes is caused by the pancreas being unable to produce the insulin the body needs to turn sugar into energy and to store excess sugar in cells. You know that type 2 diabetes often results, not from an insulin deficiency, but from insulin resistance, which is when your body cannot work with the insulin it has, making it think there is not enough insulin. In turn, the pancreas pushes out more, eventually working itself to collapse. You have been shown the way that conventional medicine treats diabetes, with medications and supplementary insulin, that more often than not cause more problems than they cure, with side effects that range from the mildly annoying to the downright dangerous. You've seen that these medications and supplemental insulin can actually make diabetes worse, by overworking the pancreas and causing it to eventually giving out, and you've learned that in this way, doctors often cause patients with type 2 diabetes to develop type 1 diabetes, rather than simply being able to manage what they have.

But then you learned that this is not the only way. There are people who are dedicated to healing a diabetic body without the use of medications, by focusing on the whole person and helping them get to a place where they can heal themselves. This can be done by using a combination of exercise, diet, and supplements, and can give a patient a much more enjoyable life than the one they would have if they were taking multiple medications.

So now what? The next step is for you to try it. If you suffer with diabetes, you know that it is not an easy road to travel. Do yourself a favor and see if the naturopathic path is easier for you than conventional medicine. You will be amazed what you can do.

Finally, if you found this book useful in anyway, a review on Amazon is always appreciated!

www.ingramcontent.com/pod-product-compliance
Lightning Source LLC
Chambersburg PA
CBHW070230290526
45789CB00004B/1561